# AUTOIMMUNE

# HEPATITIS DIET

# COOKBOOK

A comprehensive guide to nourishing your body and
supporting your liver health through the power of
delicious and nutritious recipes.

LAUREN WILLS

Autoimmune Hepatitis Diet Cookbook

# INTRODUCTION

Welcome to the Autoimmune Hepatitis Diet Cookbook! This cookbook has been carefully curated to provide you with a collection of delicious and nourishing recipes tailored specifically for individuals managing autoimmune hepatitis. Whether you have recently been diagnosed or have been living with this condition for a while, this cookbook aims to support you in maintaining a healthy and balanced diet that can positively impact your overall well-being.

Understanding the importance of diet in managing autoimmune hepatitis is crucial. The recipes included in this cookbook have been thoughtfully designed to incorporate ingredients that are known to be beneficial for individuals with this condition. The recipes focus on incorporating nutrient-dense foods, anti-inflammatory ingredients, and supportive nutrients that can help in managing symptoms and promoting liver health.

In this cookbook, you will find a wide variety of recipes spanning different meal categories, including breakfasts, salads, main courses, soups, and desserts. Each recipe is accompanied by detailed instructions, including prep time, ingredients, step-by-step directions, and nutritional values, allowing you to make informed choices about the foods you consume.

While this cookbook serves as a guide, it is essential to consult with your healthcare provider or a registered dietitian to ensure that the recipes align with your specific dietary needs and restrictions. They can provide personalized guidance based on your unique health profile and goals.

Remember, managing autoimmune hepatitis involves a holistic approach, and diet plays a significant role in supporting your health. Embracing a well-balanced diet can help minimize inflammation, support liver function, and contribute to your overall wellness.

We hope that the Autoimmune Hepatitis Diet Cookbook becomes a valuable resource in your journey toward a healthier lifestyle. May these recipes inspire you to enjoy delicious, nourishing meals that support your well-being and bring joy to your dining table, Cheers to good health!

# CHAPTER 1

## Autoimmune Hepatitis and Diet

### A. Understanding Autoimmune Hepatitis

Autoimmune Hepatitis (AIH) is a chronic liver disease characterized by inflammation and damage to the liver caused by an autoimmune response. In AIH, the body's immune system mistakenly attacks the liver cells, leading to ongoing inflammation and liver damage if left untreated. The exact cause of AIH is still unknown, but it is believed to result from a combination of genetic and environmental factors.

Autoimmune Hepatitis can affect individuals of any age, although it is more commonly diagnosed in young to middle-aged women. It is essential to diagnose and manage AIH promptly to prevent further liver damage and complications.

### B. Importance of Diet in Managing Autoimmune Hepatitis

While there is no specific diet that can cure autoimmune hepatitis, a well-balanced and healthy diet plays a crucial role in managing the condition and supporting liver health. A nutritious diet can help reduce inflammation, maintain a healthy weight, and improve overall well-being for individuals with AIH.

Proper nutrition is important to support liver function, as the liver plays a vital role in processing nutrients, detoxifying the body, and regulating metabolism. Following a healthy diet can also help manage other conditions that often coexist with AIH, such as obesity, diabetes, and high cholesterol.

C. General Dietary Guidelines for Autoimmune Hepatitis Patients

1. Limit Alcohol Consumption: Alcohol can worsen liver inflammation and damage in individuals with autoimmune hepatitis. It is essential to avoid or limit alcohol intake to protect the liver and support its healing process.

2. Reduce Sodium Intake: Excessive sodium intake can lead to fluid retention and increased blood pressure. AIH patients should aim to reduce their sodium intake by avoiding processed foods, canned soups, and salty snacks.

3. Maintain a Healthy Weight: Obesity can contribute to liver inflammation and worsen the progression of

AIH. It is important for individuals with AIH to achieve and maintain a healthy weight through a balanced diet and regular physical activity.

4. Consume a Balanced Diet: A well-balanced diet for autoimmune hepatitis should include a variety of nutrient-rich foods such as fruits, vegetables, whole grains, lean proteins, and healthy fats. These foods provide essential vitamins, minerals, antioxidants, and fiber to support overall health and liver function.

5. Choose Healthy Fats: Incorporate healthy fats into the diet, such as those found in avocados, nuts, seeds, and fatty fish like salmon. These fats provide omega-3 fatty acids, which have anti-inflammatory properties and promote heart health.

6. Limit Processed Foods: Processed foods often contain high levels of sodium, unhealthy fats, and additives that can contribute to inflammation and liver damage. It is best to minimize the consumption of processed foods and focus on whole, natural foods instead.

7. Stay Hydrated: Drinking an adequate amount of water is important for liver health and overall well-

being. Water helps to flush out toxins and supports proper digestion and metabolism.

8. Seek Individualized Guidance: While these general guidelines can be helpful, it is crucial for individuals with autoimmune hepatitis to work with a healthcare professional or a registered dietitian who specializes in liver health. They can provide personalized dietary recommendations based on individual needs, medical history, and specific goals.

By following these general dietary guidelines and working closely with healthcare professionals, individuals with autoimmune hepatitis can make informed choices to support their liver health and overall well-being. While diet alone cannot cure AIH, it can significantly contribute to the management and maintenance of a healthier lifestyle.

# CHAPTER 2

## Autoimmune Hepatitis Diet Recipes

## Breakfast Recipes

### Recipe 1: Nutrient-Packed Smoothie Bowl

Prep Time: 5 minutes

Serves: 1

**Ingredients:**

- 1 frozen banana
- 1 cup frozen mixed berries
- 1 cup spinach leaves
- 1/2 cup almond milk (or any plant-based milk)
- Toppings: sliced fresh fruits, chia seeds, shredded coconut, granola

**Directions:**

1. In a blender, combine the frozen banana, frozen mixed berries, spinach leaves, and almond milk.
2. Blend until smooth and creamy, adding more almond milk if needed to reach the desired consistency.
3. Pour the smoothie into a bowl.

4. Top with sliced fresh fruits, chia seeds, shredded coconut, and granola.

5. Serve immediately and enjoy!

**Nutritional Value per Serving:**

Calories: 320

Protein: 6g

Fat: 8g

Carbohydrates: 60g

Fiber: 10g

## Recipe 2: Gluten-Free Oatmeal with Fresh Fruits and Nuts

Prep Time: 10 minutes

Serves: 1

**Ingredients:**

- 1/2 cup gluten-free oats
- 1 cup almond milk (or any plant-based milk)
- 1/2 teaspoon cinnamon

- 1 tablespoon honey (or maple syrup for a vegan option)
- Fresh fruits (e.g., berries, sliced banana)
- Chopped nuts (e.g., almonds, walnuts)
- Optional: a sprinkle of chia seeds

**Directions:**

1. In a saucepan, combine the gluten-free oats, almond milk, and cinnamon.
2. Cook over medium heat, stirring occasionally, until the oats are tender and the mixture thickens (about 5 minutes).
3. Remove from heat and stir in the honey.
4. Transfer the oatmeal to a bowl.
5. Top with fresh fruits, chopped nuts, and a sprinkle of chia seeds if desired.
6. Serve warm and enjoy!

**Nutritional Value per Serving:**

Calories: 380

Protein: 9g

Fat: 12g

Carbohydrates: 61g

Fiber: 9g

## Recipe 3: Veggie Omelette with Spinach and Bell Peppers

Prep Time: 10 minutes

Cook Time: 10 minutes

Serves: 1

**Ingredients:**

- 2 large eggs
- 1/4 cup chopped spinach
- 1/4 cup diced bell peppers (any color)
- 2 tablespoons diced onions
- Salt and pepper to taste
- 1 teaspoon olive oil

**Directions:**

1. In a bowl, whisk the eggs until well beaten.

2. Stir in the chopped spinach, diced bell peppers, diced onions, salt, and pepper.
3. Heat olive oil in a non-stick skillet over medium heat.
4. Pour the egg mixture into the skillet and cook until the edges start to set.
5. Gently lift the edges of the omelette with a spatula and tilt the skillet to allow the uncooked eggs to flow to the edges.
6. Continue cooking until the omelette is set but still slightly runny in the center.
7. Fold the omelette in half and cook for another minute.
8. Slide the omelette onto a plate and serve hot.

**Nutritional Value per Serving:**

Calories: 180

Protein: 12g

Fat: 12g

Carbohydrates: 7g

Fiber: 2g

# Recipe 4: Anti-Inflammatory Turmeric Scrambled Eggs

Prep Time: 5 minutes

Cook Time: 5 minutes

Serves: 1

**Ingredients:**

- 2 large eggs
- 1/4 teaspoon ground turmeric
- 1/4 teaspoon ground cumin
- Salt and pepper to taste
- 1 teaspoon olive oil
- Fresh cilantro for garnish (optional)

**Directions:**

1. In a bowl, whisk the eggs until well beaten.
2. Stir in the ground turmeric, ground cumin, salt, and pepper.
3. Heat olive oil in a non-stick skillet over medium heat.
4. Pour the egg mixture into the skillet and cook, stirring frequently, until the eggs are scrambled and

cooked to your desired consistency (about 3-4 minutes).

5. Transfer the scrambled eggs to a plate.
6. Garnish with fresh cilantro if desired.
7. Serve hot.

**Nutritional Value per Serving:**

Calories: 180

Protein: 13g

Fat: 12g

Carbohydrates: 1g

Fiber: 0g

## Recipe 5: Quinoa Breakfast Bowl with Berries and Almonds

Prep Time: 10 minutes

Cook Time: 15 minutes

Serves: 1

**Ingredients:**

- 1/2 cup cooked quinoa
- 1/4 cup mixed fresh berries (e.g., strawberries, blueberries, raspberries)
- 1 tablespoon sliced almonds
- 1 tablespoon honey (or maple syrup for a vegan option)
- Optional: a sprinkle of cinnamon

**Directions:**

1. In a bowl, combine the cooked quinoa, mixed fresh berries, sliced almonds, and honey.
2. Stir well to combine.
3. Sprinkle with cinnamon if desired.
4. Serve at room temperature or chilled.

**Nutritional Value per Serving:**

Calories: 280

Protein: 9g

Fat: 7g

Carbohydrates: 47g

Fiber: 8g

## Recipe 6: Veggie-Packed Breakfast Frittata

Prep Time: 10 minutes

Cook Time: 20 minutes

Serves: 4

**Ingredients:**

- 6 large eggs
- 1/4 cup almond milk (or any plant-based milk)
- 1 cup chopped mixed vegetables (e.g., bell peppers, onions, mushrooms)
- 1 cup baby spinach leaves
- Salt and pepper to taste
- 1 tablespoon olive oil

**Directions:**

1. Preheat the oven to 350°F (175°C).
2. In a bowl, whisk the eggs until well beaten.

3. Stir in the almond milk, chopped mixed vegetables, baby spinach leaves, salt, and pepper.

4. Heat olive oil in an oven-safe skillet over medium heat.

5. Pour the egg mixture into the skillet and cook for 3-4 minutes until the edges start to set.

6. Transfer the skillet to the preheated oven and bake for 15-20 minutes or until the frittata is set and lightly golden on top.

7. Remove from the oven and let it cool slightly.

8. Slice the frittata into wedges and serve.

**Nutritional Value per Serving:**

Calories: 140

Protein: 10g

Fat: 9g

Carbohydrates: 5g

Fiber: 1g

## Lunch Recipes

### Recipe 1: Grilled Chicken and Avocado Salad

Prep Time: 15 minutes

Cook Time: 10 minutes

Serves: 2

**Ingredients:**

- 2 boneless, skinless chicken breasts
- 4 cups mixed salad greens
- 1 ripe avocado, sliced
- 1 cup cherry tomatoes, halved
- 1/4 cup sliced red onions
- Juice of 1 lemon
- 2 tablespoons olive oil
- Salt and pepper to taste

**Directions:**

1. Preheat the grill to medium-high heat.
2. Season the chicken breasts with salt and pepper.

3. Grill the chicken for 4-5 minutes per side or until cooked through. Remove from the grill and let it rest for a few minutes before slicing.

4. In a large bowl, combine the mixed salad greens, sliced avocado, cherry tomatoes, and sliced red onions.

5. In a small bowl, whisk together the lemon juice, olive oil, salt, and pepper to make the dressing.

6. Drizzle the dressing over the salad and toss gently to coat.

7. Divide the salad onto plates and top with the sliced grilled chicken.

8. Serve immediately.

**Nutritional Value per Serving:**

Calories: 320

Protein: 28g

Fat: 18g

Carbohydrates: 14g

Fiber: 8g

# Recipe 2: Roasted Vegetable Wrap with Hummus

Prep Time: 15 minutes

Cook Time: 25 minutes

Serves: 2

**Ingredients:**

- 1 cup mixed vegetables (e.g., bell peppers, zucchini, eggplant), sliced
- 1 tablespoon olive oil
- Salt and pepper to taste
- 2 whole wheat wraps or tortillas
- 1/4 cup hummus
- 1/4 cup baby spinach leaves
- 1/4 cup sliced cucumbers
- 1/4 cup sliced tomatoes
- Optional: crumbled feta cheese or goat cheese

**Directions:**

1. Preheat the oven to 400°F (200°C).
2. Toss the mixed vegetables with olive oil, salt, and pepper.

3. Spread the vegetables on a baking sheet and roast in the preheated oven for 20-25 minutes or until tender and slightly charred.
4. Warm the wraps or tortillas according to the package instructions.
5. Spread a tablespoon of hummus onto each wrap.
6. Layer the roasted vegetables, baby spinach leaves, sliced cucumbers, and sliced tomatoes on top of the hummus.
7. Optional: Sprinkle with crumbled feta cheese or goat cheese for added flavor.
8. Roll up the wraps tightly and cut in half.
9. Serve immediately or wrap tightly in foil for later.

**Nutritional Value per Serving:**

Calories: 280

Protein: 9g

Fat: 12g

Carbohydrates: 36g

Fiber: 6g

## Recipe 3: Sweet Potato and Black Bean Bowl

Prep Time: 15 minutes

Cook Time: 30 minutes

Serves: 2

**Ingredients:**

- 2 medium sweet potatoes, peeled and diced
- 1 tablespoon olive oil
- 1 teaspoon ground cumin
- 1/2 teaspoon chili powder
- Salt and pepper to taste
- 1 cup cooked black beans
- 1 cup cooked quinoa
- 1/4 cup chopped fresh cilantro
- Juice of 1 lime
- Optional toppings: sliced avocado, diced tomatoes, Greek yogurt (for serving)

**Directions:**

1. Preheat the oven to 425°F (220°C).

2. Toss the diced sweet potatoes with olive oil, ground cumin, chili powder, salt, and pepper.

3. Spread the sweet potatoes on a baking sheet and roast in the preheated oven for 25-30 minutes or until tender and golden.

4. In a large bowl, combine the roasted sweet potatoes, cooked black beans, cooked quinoa, chopped fresh cilantro, and lime juice.

5. Toss gently to combine.

6. Divide the mixture into bowls.

7. Optional: Top with sliced avocado, diced tomatoes, and a dollop of Greek yogurt.

8. Serve warm.

**Nutritional Value per Serving:**

Calories: 380

Protein: 12g

Fat: 8g

Carbohydrates: 67g

Fiber: 12g

## Dinner Recipes

### Recipe 1: Baked Cod with Lemon and Dill

Prep Time: 10 minutes

Cook Time: 15 minutes

Serves: 2

**Ingredients:**

- 2 cod fillets
- 1 lemon, sliced
- 2 tablespoons fresh dill, chopped
- 2 tablespoons olive oil
- Salt and pepper to taste

**Directions:**

1. Preheat the oven to 400°F (200°C).
2. Place the cod fillets in a baking dish.
3. Drizzle the olive oil over the fillets and season with salt and pepper.
4. Arrange the lemon slices on top of the fillets and sprinkle with fresh dill.

5. Bake in the preheated oven for 12-15 minutes or until the cod is opaque and flakes easily with a fork.
6. Remove from the oven and serve hot.

**Nutritional Value per Serving:**

Calories: 220

Protein: 30g

Fat: 10g

Carbohydrates: 2g

Fiber: 0g

### Recipe 2: Quinoa-Stuffed Bell Peppers

Prep Time: 15 minutes

Cook Time: 35 minutes

Serves: 4

**Ingredients:**

- 4 bell peppers (any color), tops removed and seeds removed

- 1 cup cooked quinoa
- 1/2 cup diced tomatoes
- 1/2 cup black beans, rinsed and drained
- 1/2 cup corn kernels
- 1/4 cup chopped fresh parsley
- 1/4 cup shredded cheese (e.g., cheddar, mozzarella)
- 1 teaspoon olive oil
- Salt and pepper to taste

**Directions:**

1. Preheat the oven to 375°F (190°C).
2. Place the bell peppers in a baking dish, cut-side up.
3. In a bowl, combine the cooked quinoa, diced tomatoes, black beans, corn kernels, chopped fresh parsley, shredded cheese, olive oil, salt, and pepper.
4. Spoon the quinoa mixture into the bell peppers, filling them evenly.
5. Cover the baking dish with foil and bake in the preheated oven for 25 minutes.
6. Remove the foil and bake for an additional 10 minutes or until the peppers are tender and the filling is heated through.

7. Remove from the oven and let it cool slightly before serving.

**Nutritional Value per Serving:**

Calories: 220

Protein: 9g

Fat: 6g

Carbohydrates: 37g

Fiber: 7g

**Recipe 3: Stir-Fried Tofu with Mixed Vegetables**

Prep Time: 15 minutes

Cook Time: 10 minutes

Serves: 2

**Ingredients:**

- 8 ounces firm tofu, drained and cubed
- 1 tablespoon soy sauce (or tamari for a gluten-free option)

- 1 tablespoon hoisin sauce
- 1 tablespoon sesame oil
- 1 tablespoon olive oil
- 2 cloves garlic, minced
- 1 cup mixed vegetables (e.g., broccoli, bell peppers, carrots), sliced
- Salt and pepper to taste
- Optional toppings: sliced green onions, sesame seeds

**Directions:**

1. In a bowl, combine the soy sauce, hoisin sauce, and sesame oil.
2. Add the cubed tofu to the bowl and toss gently to coat. Let it marinate for 10 minutes.
3. Heat olive oil in a large skillet or wok over medium-high heat.
4. Add the minced garlic and stir-fry for 1 minute until fragrant.
5. Add the mixed vegetables and stir-fry for 3-4 minutes or until they are tender-crisp.
6. Push the vegetables to one side of the skillet and add the marinated tofu.

7. Cook the tofu for 3-4 minutes, flipping occasionally, until it is browned and heated through.
8. Season with salt and pepper to taste.
9. Optional: Top with sliced green onions and sesame seeds for garnish.
10. Serve hot.

**Nutritional Value per Serving:**

Calories: 250

Protein: 15g

Fat: 17g

Carbohydrates: 12g

Fiber: 3g

## Appetizers and Snacks

### Recipe 1: Baked Sweet Potato Fries with Guacamole

Prep Time: 15 minutes

Cook Time: 25 minutes

Serves: 2

**Ingredients:**

- 2 medium sweet potatoes, cut into fries
- 1 tablespoon olive oil
- 1 teaspoon paprika
- 1/2 teaspoon garlic powder
- Salt and pepper to taste
- 1 ripe avocado
- Juice of 1 lime
- 1 tablespoon chopped fresh cilantro
- Optional toppings: sliced jalapeños, diced tomatoes

**Directions:**

1. Preheat the oven to 425°F (220°C).

2. In a bowl, toss the sweet potato fries with olive oil, paprika, garlic powder, salt, and pepper until evenly coated.

3. Spread the sweet potato fries on a baking sheet in a single layer.

4. Bake in the preheated oven for 20-25 minutes or until the fries are crispy and golden brown, flipping them halfway through.

5. While the fries are baking, prepare the guacamole by mashing the avocado with lime juice and chopped fresh cilantro.

6. Season the guacamole with salt and pepper to taste.

7. Once the sweet potato fries are done, remove them from the oven and let them cool slightly.

8. Serve the baked sweet potato fries with the guacamole on the side.

9. Optional: Top the guacamole with sliced jalapeños and diced tomatoes for added flavor.

**Nutritional Value per Serving:**

Calories: 320

Protein: 5g

Fat: 18g

Carbohydrates: 38g

Fiber: 9g

## Recipe 2: Cucumber and Carrot Sticks with Hummus

Prep Time: 10 minutes

Serves: 2

**Ingredients:**

- 1 cucumber, cut into sticks
- 2 carrots, cut into sticks
- 1/2 cup hummus

**Directions:**

1. Wash and cut the cucumber and carrots into sticks.
2. Arrange the cucumber and carrot sticks on a serving platter.
3. Serve the sticks with a bowl of hummus for dipping.

**Nutritional Value per Serving:**

Calories: 120

Protein: 5g

Fat: 6g

Carbohydrates: 15g

Fiber: 7g

## Recipe 3: Quinoa and Vegetable Sushi Rolls

Prep Time: 30 minutes

Cook Time: 20 minutes

Serves: 4

**Ingredients:**

- 4 nori seaweed sheets
- 2 cups cooked quinoa, cooled
- 1 cup mixed vegetables (e.g., cucumber, carrots, bell peppers), julienned
- 2 tablespoons rice vinegar
- 1 tablespoon soy sauce (or tamari for a gluten-free option)

- 1 tablespoon sesame oil
- Optional: pickled ginger, wasabi, soy sauce (for serving)

**Directions:**

1. Place a nori seaweed sheet on a sushi mat or a clean kitchen towel.
2. Spread a quarter of the cooked quinoa evenly over the nori, leaving a 1-inch border at the top.
3. Arrange a quarter of the julienned vegetables on top of the quinoa.
4. Drizzle the rice vinegar, soy sauce, and sesame oil over the vegetables.
5. Starting from the bottom, tightly roll the nori sheet, using the sushi mat or towel to help you.
6. Wet the top border of the nori sheet with water to seal the roll.
7. Repeat the process with the remaining ingredients to make three more rolls.
8. Using a sharp knife, slice each roll into bite-sized pieces.

9. Serve the sushi rolls with pickled ginger, wasabi, and soy sauce on the side.

**Nutritional Value per Serving:**

Calories: 200

Protein: 6g

Fat: 6g

Carbohydrates: 32g

Fiber: 5g

## Recipe 4: Quinoa Salad with Roasted Vegetables

Prep Time: 15 minutes

Cook Time: 25 minutes

Serves: 4

**Ingredients:**

- 1 cup cooked quinoa, cooled
- 2 cups mixed vegetables (e.g., bell peppers, zucchini, eggplant), diced

- 2 tablespoons olive oil
- 1 teaspoon dried herbs (e.g., thyme, oregano)
- Salt and pepper to taste
- Juice of 1 lemon
- 2 tablespoons chopped fresh parsley
- Optional toppings: crumbled feta cheese, toasted nuts or seeds

**Directions:**

1. Preheat the oven to 400°F (200°C).
2. Toss the diced vegetables with olive oil, dried herbs, salt, and pepper.
3. Spread the vegetables on a baking sheet in a single layer.
4. Roast in the preheated oven for 20-25 minutes or until the vegetables are tender and slightly charred.
5. In a large bowl, combine the cooked quinoa, roasted vegetables, lemon juice, and chopped fresh parsley.
6. Toss gently to combine.
7. Optional: Sprinkle with crumbled feta cheese or toasted nuts/seeds for added flavor.

8. Serve the quinoa salad at room temperature or chilled.

**Nutritional Value per Serving:**

Calories: 220

Protein: 6g

Fat: 9g

Carbohydrates: 30g

Fiber: 6g

## Recipe 5: Baked Sweet Potato Chips with Guacamole

Prep Time: 10 minutes

Cook Time: 20 minutes

Serves: 2

**Ingredients:**

- 2 medium sweet potatoes, thinly sliced
- 1 tablespoon olive oil

- Salt and pepper to taste
- 1 ripe avocado
- Juice of 1 lime
- 1 tablespoon chopped fresh cilantro
- Optional toppings: sliced jalapeños, diced tomatoes

**Directions:**

1. Preheat the oven to 400°F (200°C).
2. Toss the sweet potato slices with olive oil, salt, and pepper until evenly coated.
3. Arrange the sweet potato slices on a baking sheet in a single layer.
4. Bake in the preheated oven for 15-20 minutes or until the chips are crispy and lightly browned, flipping them halfway through.
5. While the chips are baking, prepare the guacamole by mashing the avocado with lime juice and chopped fresh cilantro.
6. Season the guacamole with salt and pepper to taste.
7. Once the sweet potato chips are done, remove them from the oven and let them cool slightly.

8. Serve the baked sweet potato chips with the guacamole on the side.

9. Optional: Top the guacamole with sliced jalapeños and diced tomatoes for added flavor.

**Nutritional Value per Serving:**

Calories: 280

Protein: 4g

Fat: 16g

Carbohydrates: 32g

Fiber: 7g

## Recipe 6: Hummus with Fresh Vegetables

Prep Time: 10 minutes

Serves: 2

**Ingredients:**

1 cup canned chickpeas, rinsed and drained

2 tablespoons tahini

2 tablespoons olive oil

Juice of 1 lemon

1 clove garlic, minced

Salt and pepper to taste

Assorted fresh vegetables (e.g., bell peppers, cucumbers, carrots), cut into sticks

**Directions:**

In a food processor, combine the chickpeas, tahini, olive oil, lemon juice, minced garlic, salt, and pepper.

Blend until smooth and creamy, adding a little water if needed to achieve the desired consistency.

Transfer the hummus to a serving bowl.

Serve the hummus with assorted fresh vegetables for dipping.

**Nutritional Value per Serving:**

Calories: 250

Protein: 8g

Fat: 16g

Carbohydrates: 22g

Fiber: 6g

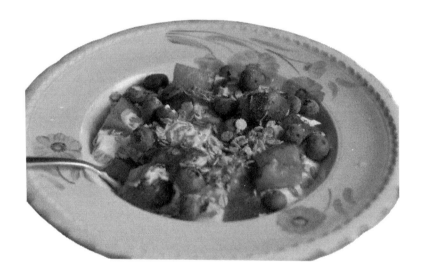

CEREALS & BLUBERRIES

## Main Course

### Recipe 1: Grilled Salmon with Quinoa and Steamed Vegetables

Prep Time: 15 minutes

Cook Time: 15 minutes

Serves: 2

**Ingredients:**

- 2 salmon fillets
- 1 tablespoon olive oil
- Juice of 1 lemon
- Salt and pepper to taste
- 1 cup cooked quinoa
- 2 cups mixed steamed vegetables (e.g., broccoli, carrots, cauliflower)

**Directions:**

1. Preheat the grill to medium heat.
2. Brush the salmon fillets with olive oil and lemon juice.
3. Season with salt and pepper to taste.

4. Place the salmon fillets on the grill and cook for about 6-8 minutes per side, or until the fish flakes easily with a fork.

5. While the salmon is grilling, prepare the quinoa according to the package instructions.

6. Steam the mixed vegetables until tender but still crisp.

7. Serve the grilled salmon on a bed of cooked quinoa with a side of steamed vegetables.

**Nutritional Value per Serving:**

Calories: 400

Protein: 30g

Fat: 20g

Carbohydrates: 25g

Fiber: 5g

**Recipe 2: Baked Chicken Breast with Roasted Brussels Sprouts**

Prep Time: 15 minutes

Cook Time: 25 minutes

Serves: 2

**Ingredients:**

- 2 chicken breast halves
- 1 tablespoon olive oil
- 1 teaspoon dried herbs (e.g., rosemary, thyme)
- Salt and pepper to taste
- 2 cups Brussels sprouts, trimmed and halved
- 1 tablespoon balsamic vinegar
- Optional: lemon wedges for serving

**Directions:**

1. Preheat the oven to 400°F (200°C).
2. Place the chicken breast halves on a baking sheet.
3. Drizzle the chicken breasts with olive oil and sprinkle with dried herbs, salt, and pepper.
4. In a separate bowl, toss the Brussels sprouts with olive oil, balsamic vinegar, salt, and pepper.
5. Spread the Brussels sprouts on the baking sheet around the chicken breasts.

6. Bake in the preheated oven for 20-25 minutes or until the chicken is cooked through and the Brussels sprouts are tender and caramelized.
7. Remove from the oven and let it rest for a few minutes before serving.
8. Serve the baked chicken breast with roasted Brussels sprouts and optional lemon wedges.

**Nutritional Value per Serving:**

Calories: 350

Protein: 40g

Fat: 12g

Carbohydrates: 20g

Fiber: 8g

## Recipe 3: Lentil Stew with Brown Rice

Prep Time: 15 minutes

Cook Time: 40 minutes

Serves: 4

**Ingredients:**

- 1 cup brown lentils, rinsed and drained
- 1 tablespoon olive oil
- 1 onion, chopped
- 2 carrots, diced
- 2 celery stalks, diced
- 3 cloves garlic, minced
- 1 teaspoon ground cumin
- 1 teaspoon paprika
- 4 cups vegetable broth
- 1 bay leaf
- Salt and pepper to taste
- 2 cups cooked brown rice
- Optional toppings: chopped fresh parsley, lemon wedges

**Directions:**

1. In a large pot, heat olive oil over medium heat.
2. Add the onion, carrots, and celery, and sauté for 5 minutes until the vegetables start to soften.

3. Add the minced garlic, cumin, and paprika, and sauté for another minute until fragrant.
4. Add the rinsed lentils, vegetable broth, and bay leaf to the pot.
5. Season with salt and pepper to taste.
6. Bring the stew to a boil, then reduce the heat to low and simmer for 30-35 minutes or until the lentils are tender.
7. Remove the bay leaf and adjust the seasonings if needed.
8. Serve the lentil stew over cooked brown rice.
9. Optional: Garnish with chopped fresh parsley and serve with lemon wedges on the side.

**Nutritional Value per Serving:**

Calories: 300

Protein: 15g

Fat: 5g

Carbohydrates: 55g

Fiber: 10g

## Side Dishes

### Recipe 1: Roasted Brussels sprouts with Balsamic Glaze

Prep Time: 10 minutes

Cook Time: 25 minutes

Serves: 4

**Ingredients:**

- 1 pound Brussels sprouts, trimmed and halved
- 2 tablespoons olive oil
- Salt and pepper to taste
- 2 tablespoons balsamic glaze

**Directions:**

1. Preheat the oven to 400°F (200°C).
2. In a bowl, toss the Brussels sprouts with olive oil, salt, and pepper until evenly coated.
3. Spread the Brussels sprouts on a baking sheet in a single layer.
4. Roast in the preheated oven for 20-25 minutes or until the Brussels sprouts are tender and caramelized.

5. Remove from the oven and drizzle with balsamic glaze.
6. Toss gently to coat.
7. Serve the roasted Brussels sprouts as a side dish.

**Nutritional Value per Serving:**

Calories: 100

Protein: 4g

Fat: 6g

Carbohydrates: 10g

Fiber: 4g

## Recipe 2: Mashed Cauliflower with Herbs

Prep Time: 10 minutes

Cook Time: 15 minutes

Serves: 4

**Ingredients:**

- 1 large head cauliflower, cut into florets

- 2 tablespoons butter or olive oil
- 2 cloves garlic, minced
- 1/4 cup milk (or non-dairy alternative)
- 1 tablespoon chopped fresh herbs (e.g., parsley, thyme)
- Salt and pepper to taste

**Directions:**

1. Steam the cauliflower florets until tender.
2. In a saucepan, melt the butter or heat the olive oil over medium heat.
3. Add the minced garlic and sauté for 1-2 minutes until fragrant.
4. Transfer the steamed cauliflower to the saucepan and mash with a potato masher or blend in a food processor until smooth.
5. Stir in the milk and chopped fresh herbs.
6. Season with salt and pepper to taste.
7. Cook for another 2-3 minutes until heated through.
8. Serve the mashed cauliflower as a healthy alternative to traditional mashed potatoes.

**Nutritional Value per Serving:**

Calories: 70

Protein: 3g

Fat: 4g

Carbohydrates: 8g

Fiber: 3g

## Recipe 3: Sautéed Spinach with Garlic and Lemon

Prep Time: 5 minutes

Cook Time: 5 minutes

Serves: 4

**Ingredients:**

- 1 tablespoon olive oil
- 2 cloves garlic, minced
- 8 cups fresh spinach leaves
- Juice of 1 lemon
- Salt and pepper to taste

**Directions:**

1. In a large skillet, heat the olive oil over medium heat.
2. Add the minced garlic and sauté for 1 minute until fragrant.
3. Add the spinach leaves to the skillet and toss gently until wilted.
4. Drizzle the lemon juice over the spinach.
5. Season with salt and pepper to taste.
6. Cook for another 1-2 minutes until heated through.
7. Serve the sautéed spinach as a nutritious side dish.

**Nutritional Value per Serving:**

Calories: 40

Protein: 2g

Fat: 3g

Carbohydrates: 3g

Fiber: 2g

### Recipe 4: Roasted Garlic Cauliflower Mash

Prep Time: 10 minutes

Cook Time: 40 minutes

Serves: 4

**Ingredients:**

- 1 large head cauliflower, cut into florets
- 2 tablespoons olive oil
- 4 cloves garlic, peeled
- Salt and pepper to taste
- 1/4 cup vegetable broth (or more as needed)

**Directions:**

1. Preheat the oven to 400°F (200°C).
2. Place the cauliflower florets and peeled garlic cloves on a baking sheet.
3. Drizzle with olive oil and season with salt and pepper to taste.
4. Roast in the preheated oven for 30-35 minutes or until the cauliflower is tender and golden.
5. Transfer the roasted cauliflower and garlic to a food processor.

6. Blend until smooth, adding vegetable broth as needed to achieve the desired consistency.
7. Season with additional salt and pepper if desired.
8. Serve the roasted garlic cauliflower mash as a flavorful and healthy side dish.

**Nutritional Value per Serving:**

Calories: 80

Protein: 3g

Fat: 5g

Carbohydrates: 8g

Fiber: 4g

## Recipe 5: Steamed Broccoli with Lemon and Almonds

Prep Time: 10 minutes

Cook Time: 5 minutes

Serves: 4

**Ingredients:**

- 4 cups broccoli florets
- 1 tablespoon olive oil
- Juice of 1 lemon
- Zest of 1 lemon
- Salt and pepper to taste
- 2 tablespoons sliced almonds, toasted

**Directions:**

1. Steam the broccoli florets until crisp-tender.
2. In a small bowl, whisk together the olive oil, lemon juice, lemon zest, salt, and pepper.
3. Drizzle the lemon dressing over the steamed broccoli.
4. Toss gently to coat.
5. Sprinkle with toasted sliced almonds.
6. Serve the steamed broccoli as a nutritious and vibrant side dish.

**Nutritional Value per Serving:**

Calories: 60

Protein: 3g

Fat: 4g

Carbohydrates: 6g

Fiber: 3g

## Recipe 6: Quinoa Pilaf with Mixed Vegetables

Prep Time: 10 minutes

Cook Time: 20 minutes

Serves: 4

**Ingredients:**

- 1 cup quinoa, rinsed
- 2 cups vegetable broth
- 1 tablespoon olive oil
- 1 onion, chopped
- 2 cloves garlic, minced
- 1 carrot, diced
- 1 zucchini, diced
- 1 red bell pepper, diced
- Salt and pepper to taste

- 2 tablespoons chopped fresh herbs (e.g., parsley, basil)

**Directions:**

1. In a saucepan, combine the quinoa and vegetable broth.
2. Bring to a boil, then reduce the heat to low, cover, and simmer for 15-20 minutes or until the quinoa is tender and the broth is absorbed.
3. In a separate skillet, heat the olive oil over medium heat.
4. Add the chopped onion and minced garlic, and sauté for 2-3 minutes until softened.
5. Add the diced carrot, zucchini, and red bell pepper to the skillet.
6. Sauté for another 5 minutes until the vegetables are tender-crisp.
7. Season with salt and pepper to taste.
8. Fluff the cooked quinoa with a fork and transfer it to the skillet with the sautéed vegetables.
9. Stir in the chopped fresh herbs and mix well.
10. Cook for another 2-3 minutes until heated through.

11. Serve the quinoa pilaf with mixed vegetables as a wholesome and flavorful side dish.

**Nutritional Value per Serving:**

Calories: 180

Protein: 5g

Fat: 5g

Carbohydrates: 30g

Fiber: 5g

## Soups and Stews

### Recipe 1: Healing Turmeric Ginger Soup

Prep Time: 10 minutes

Cook Time: 30 minutes

Serves: 4

**Ingredients:**

- 1 tablespoon olive oil
- 1 onion, chopped
- 2 cloves garlic, minced
- 1-inch piece of fresh ginger, grated
- 1 teaspoon ground turmeric
- 4 cups vegetable broth
- 2 carrots, diced
- 2 stalks celery, diced
- 1 cup cauliflower florets
- 1 cup diced tomatoes (canned or fresh)
- Salt and pepper to taste
- Optional toppings: fresh cilantro, lime wedges

**Directions:**

1. Heat olive oil in a large pot over medium heat.
2. Add the chopped onion, minced garlic, and grated ginger. Sauté for 2-3 minutes until fragrant.
3. Stir in the ground turmeric and cook for another minute.
4. Add the vegetable broth, diced carrots, celery, cauliflower florets, and diced tomatoes to the pot.
5. Season with salt and pepper to taste.
6. Bring the soup to a boil, then reduce the heat to low and simmer for 20-25 minutes until the vegetables are tender.
7. Remove from heat and let the soup cool slightly.
8. Using an immersion blender or countertop blender, puree the soup until smooth.
9. Reheat the soup if needed.
10. Serve the healing turmeric ginger soup hot, garnished with fresh cilantro and lime wedges if desired.

**Nutritional Value per Serving:**

Calories: 120

Protein: 3g

Fat: 4g

Carbohydrates: 20g

Fiber: 5g

**Recipe 2: Lentil and Vegetable Stew**

Prep Time: 10 minutes

Cook Time: 35 minutes

Serves: 4

**Ingredients:**

- 1 tablespoon olive oil
- 1 onion, chopped
- 2 cloves garlic, minced
- 2 carrots, diced
- 2 celery stalks, diced
- 1 cup diced tomatoes (canned or fresh)
- 1 cup green or brown lentils, rinsed
- 4 cups vegetable broth

- 1 teaspoon dried thyme
- Salt and pepper to taste
- Optional toppings: chopped fresh parsley

**Directions:**

1. Heat olive oil in a large pot over medium heat.
2. Add the chopped onion, minced garlic, diced carrots, and diced celery. Sauté for 5 minutes until the vegetables start to soften.
3. Stir in the diced tomatoes and cook for another 2 minutes.
4. Add the rinsed lentils, vegetable broth, dried thyme, salt, and pepper to the pot.
5. Bring the stew to a boil, then reduce the heat to low and simmer for 30 minutes or until the lentils are tender.
6. Adjust the seasonings if needed.
7. Serve the lentil and vegetable stew hot, garnished with chopped fresh parsley if desired.

**Nutritional Value per Serving:**

Calories: 250

Protein: 13g

Fat: 4g

Carbohydrates: 45g

Fiber: 12g

## Recipe 3: Chicken and Vegetable Bone Broth Soup

Prep Time: 10 minutes

Cook Time: 2 hours

Serves: 4

**Ingredients:**

- 1 whole chicken, organic and free-range if possible
- 8 cups water
- 2 carrots, chopped
- 2 celery stalks, chopped
- 1 onion, chopped
- 3 cloves garlic, minced
- 1-inch piece of fresh ginger, grated
- 1 bay leaf

- Salt and pepper to taste

- Optional toppings: chopped fresh parsley, lemon wedges

**Directions:**

1. Place the whole chicken, water, chopped carrots, chopped celery, chopped onion, minced garlic, grated ginger, bay leaf, salt, and pepper in a large pot.
2. Bring the pot to a boil over high heat.
3. Reduce the heat to low, cover, and simmer for 1.5 to 2 hours until the chicken is cooked through and tender.
4. Remove the chicken from the pot and set aside to cool.
5. Strain the broth into a separate pot or large bowl, discarding the vegetables and bay leaf.
6. Once the chicken has cooled, remove the meat from the bones and shred or chop it into bite-sized pieces.
7. Return the strained broth to the pot and add the shredded chicken.
8. Bring the soup to a simmer over medium heat and cook for another 10 minutes.

9. Adjust the seasonings if needed.

10. Serve the chicken and vegetable bone broth soup hot, garnished with chopped fresh parsley and lemon wedges if desired.

**Nutritional Value per Serving:**

Calories: 200

Protein: 20g

Fat: 8g

Carbohydrates: 8g

Fiber: 2g

## Salads

### Recipe 1: Kale Salad with Citrus Vinaigrette

Prep Time: 15 minutes

Serves: 4

**Ingredients:**

- 8 cups kale, stems removed and leaves chopped
- 1 cup cherry tomatoes, halved
- 1/4 cup sliced almonds, toasted
- 1/4 cup dried cranberries
- 1/4 cup grated Parmesan cheese (optional)

For the Citrus Vinaigrette:

- Juice of 1 orange
- Juice of 1 lemon
- 2 tablespoons extra-virgin olive oil
- 1 teaspoon Dijon mustard
- Salt and pepper to taste

**Directions:**

1. In a large salad bowl, combine the chopped kale, cherry tomatoes, sliced almonds, dried cranberries, and grated Parmesan cheese (if using).
2. In a separate small bowl, whisk together the orange juice, lemon juice, olive oil, Dijon mustard, salt, and pepper to make the citrus vinaigrette.
3. Drizzle the citrus vinaigrette over the kale salad.
4. Toss gently to coat the salad with the dressing.
5. Allow the salad to marinate for 10-15 minutes to let the flavors meld together.
6. Serve the kale salad with citrus vinaigrette as a refreshing and nutritious side dish.

**Nutritional Value per Serving:**

Calories: 150

Protein: 6g

Fat: 9g

Carbohydrates: 16g

Fiber: 4g

## Recipe 2: Mediterranean Quinoa Salad

Prep Time: 15 minutes

Cook Time: 15 minutes

Serves: 4

**Ingredients:**

- 1 cup quinoa
- 2 cups water
- 1 cup cucumber, diced
- 1 cup cherry tomatoes, halved
- 1/2 cup Kalamata olives, pitted and halved
- 1/2 cup crumbled feta cheese
- 1/4 cup red onion, finely chopped
- 1/4 cup chopped fresh parsley
- 2 tablespoons extra-virgin olive oil
- Juice of 1 lemon
- Salt and pepper to taste

**Directions:**

1. Rinse the quinoa under cold water in a fine-mesh sieve.

2. In a medium saucepan, bring the water to a boil.

3. Add the rinsed quinoa to the boiling water, reduce the heat to low, cover, and simmer for 15 minutes or until the water is absorbed and the quinoa is tender.

4. Remove the cooked quinoa from heat and let it cool.

5. In a large salad bowl, combine the cooled quinoa, diced cucumber, cherry tomatoes, Kalamata olives, crumbled feta cheese, red onion, and chopped fresh parsley.

6. In a separate small bowl, whisk together the olive oil, lemon juice, salt, and pepper to make the dressing.

7. Drizzle the dressing over the quinoa salad.

8. Toss gently to coat the salad with the dressing.

9. Serve the Mediterranean quinoa salad as a vibrant and flavorful side dish or light meal.

**Nutritional Value per Serving:**

Calories: 300

Protein: 10g

Fat: 14g

Carbohydrates: 36g

Fiber: 5g

## Recipe 3: Avocado and Tomato Salad with Balsamic Dressing

Prep Time: 10 minutes

Serves: 4

**Ingredients:**

- 2 avocados, diced
- 2 cups cherry tomatoes, halved
- 1/4 cup red onion, finely chopped
- 2 tablespoons chopped fresh basil
- 2 tablespoons extra-virgin olive oil
- 1 tablespoon balsamic vinegar
- Salt and pepper to taste

**Directions:**

1. In a large salad bowl, combine the diced avocados, cherry tomatoes, red onion, and chopped fresh basil.

2. In a separate small bowl, whisk together the olive oil, balsamic vinegar, salt, and pepper to make the dressing.

3. Drizzle the dressing over the avocado and tomato salad.

4. Gently toss to coat the salad with the dressing.

5. Serve the avocado and tomato salad with balsamic dressing as a refreshing and satisfying side dish.

**Nutritional Value per Serving:**

Calories: 200

Protein: 3g

Fat: 17g

Carbohydrates: 12g

Fiber: 7g

## Desserts

### Recipe 1: Coconut Flour Blueberry Muffins

Prep Time: 10 minutes

Cook Time: 25 minutes

Makes: 12 muffins

**Ingredients:**

- 1/2 cup coconut flour
- 1/2 teaspoon baking powder
- 1/4 teaspoon salt
- 4 eggs
- 1/4 cup coconut oil, melted
- 1/4 cup honey or maple syrup
- 1 teaspoon vanilla extract
- 1 cup blueberries (fresh or frozen)

**Directions:**

1. Preheat the oven to 350°F (175°C) and line a muffin tin with paper liners.
2. In a bowl, whisk together the coconut flour, baking powder, and salt.

3. In a separate bowl, beat the eggs, coconut oil, honey or maple syrup, and vanilla extract until well combined.
4. Add the dry ingredients to the wet ingredients and mix until smooth.
5. Gently fold in the blueberries.
6. Divide the batter evenly among the prepared muffin cups.
7. Bake for 20-25 minutes, or until a toothpick inserted into the center of a muffin comes out clean.
8. Allow the muffins to cool in the pan for a few minutes, then transfer them to a wire rack to cool completely.
9. Enjoy these delicious coconut flour blueberry muffins as a healthy and satisfying treat.

**Nutritional Value per serving (1 muffin):**

Calories: 110

Protein: 3g

Fat: 7g

Carbohydrates: 9g

Fiber: 3g

## Recipe 2: Almond Flour Banana Bread

Prep Time: 15 minutes

Cook Time: 45 minutes

Makes: 1 loaf

**Ingredients:**

- 2 cups almond flour
- 1 teaspoon baking powder
- 1/2 teaspoon baking soda
- 1/4 teaspoon salt
- 1 teaspoon ground cinnamon
- 3 ripe bananas, mashed
- 3 eggs
- 1/4 cup honey or maple syrup
- 1/4 cup coconut oil, melted
- 1 teaspoon vanilla extract

**Directions:**

1. Preheat the oven to 350°F (175°C) and grease a loaf pan.

2. In a large bowl, whisk together the almond flour, baking powder, baking soda, salt, and cinnamon.

3. In a separate bowl, mix the mashed bananas, eggs, honey or maple syrup, melted coconut oil, and vanilla extract until well combined.

4. Add the wet ingredients to the dry ingredients and stir until just combined.

5. Pour the batter into the greased loaf pan.

6. Bake for 40-45 minutes, or until a toothpick inserted into the center of the bread comes out clean.

7. Allow the banana bread to cool in the pan for 10 minutes, then transfer it to a wire rack to cool completely.

8. Slice and serve the almond flour banana bread as a delightful and nutritious treat.

**Nutritional Value per Serving (1 slice):**

Calories: 200

Protein: 6g

Fat: 15g

Carbohydrates: 13g

Fiber: 3g


## Recipe 3: Dark Chocolate Avocado Mousse

Prep Time: 10 minutes

Chill Time: 2 hours

Serves: 4

**Ingredients:**

- 2 ripe avocados
- 1/4 cup unsweetened cocoa powder
- 1/4 cup maple syrup or honey
- 1/4 cup almond milk (or any non-dairy milk)
- 1 teaspoon vanilla extract
- Optional toppings: dark chocolate shavings, fresh berries, chopped nuts

## Directions:

1. Cut the avocados in half, remove the pits, and scoop the flesh into a blender or food processor.

2. Add the cocoa powder, maple syrup or honey, almond milk, and vanilla extract to the blender.

3. Blend until smooth and creamy, scraping down the sides as needed.

4. Taste and adjust the sweetness if desired.

5. Transfer the mousse to serving dishes or ramekins.

6. Cover and refrigerate for at least 2 hours to allow the mousse to set.

7. Before serving, garnish with dark chocolate shavings, fresh berries, or chopped nuts if desired.

8. Enjoy this rich and indulgent dark chocolate avocado mousse as a guilt-free dessert.

## Nutritional Value per Serving:

Calories: 180

Protein: 3g

Fat: 14g

Carbohydrates: 15g

Fiber: 7g

**Recipe 4: Berry Chia Pudding**

Prep Time: 10 minutes

Chill Time: 2-4 hours

Serves: 2

**Ingredients:**

- 1 cup unsweetened almond milk (or any non-dairy milk)
- 1/4 cup chia seeds
- 1 tablespoon maple syrup or honey
- 1/2 teaspoon vanilla extract
- 1/2 cup mixed berries (such as strawberries, blueberries, raspberries)

**Directions:**

1. In a bowl, whisk together the almond milk, chia seeds, maple syrup or honey, and vanilla extract.
2. Let the mixture sit for 5 minutes, then whisk again to break up any clumps of chia seeds.

3. Cover the bowl and refrigerate for 2-4 hours, or overnight, until the chia pudding has thickened.
4. Stir the chia pudding well before serving to evenly distribute the chia seeds.
5. Divide the chia pudding into serving glasses or bowls.
6. Top with mixed berries.
7. Serve the berry chia pudding as a nutritious and satisfying breakfast or snack.

**Nutritional Value per Serving:**

Calories: 150

Protein: 5g

Fat: 9g

Carbohydrates: 15g

Fiber: 9g

## Recipe 5: Baked Apples with Cinnamon and Walnuts

Prep Time: 10 minutes

Cook Time: 30 minutes

Serves: 4

**Ingredients:**

- 4 apples (such as Granny Smith or Honeycrisp)
- 1/4 cup chopped walnuts
- 2 tablespoons maple syrup or honey
- 1 teaspoon ground cinnamon
- Optional toppings: Greek yogurt, drizzle of honey

**Directions:**

1. Preheat the oven to 375°F (190°C) and line a baking dish with parchment paper.
2. Core the apples using an apple corer or a small knife, leaving the bottoms intact.
3. In a small bowl, combine the chopped walnuts, maple syrup or honey, and ground cinnamon.

4. Stuff each cored apple with the walnut mixture, pressing it down gently.
5. Place the stuffed apples in the prepared baking dish.
6. Bake for 25-30 minutes, or until the apples are tender and the filling is lightly browned.
7. Remove the baked apples from the oven and let them cool for a few minutes.
8. Serve the baked apples with cinnamon and walnuts as a comforting and nourishing dessert.
9. Optional: Top with a dollop of Greek yogurt and drizzle with honey for added creaminess and sweetness.

**Nutritional Value per Serving:**

Calories: 180

Protein: 3g

Fat: 6g

Carbohydrates: 33g

Fiber: 6g

Beverages

## Recipe 1: Green Detox Smoothie

Prep Time: 5 minutes

Serves: 1

**Ingredients:**

- 1 cup spinach
- 1/2 cucumber, peeled and chopped
- 1/2 green apple, cored and chopped
- 1/2 banana
- 1/2 lemon, juiced
- 1/2 cup coconut water or almond milk
- Optional: a handful of ice cubes

**Directions:**

1. In a blender, combine the spinach, cucumber, green apple, banana, lemon juice, and coconut water or almond milk.
2. Blend on high speed until smooth and creamy.
3. If desired, add a handful of ice cubes and blend again until chilled.

4. Pour the green detox smoothie into a glass and enjoy as a refreshing and nutritious way to start your day.

**Nutritional Value per Serving:**

Calories: 150

Protein: 3g

Fat: 1g

Carbohydrates: 35g

Fiber: 7g

**Recipe 2: Anti-Inflammatory Golden Milk**

Prep Time: 5 minutes

Cook Time: 5 minutes

Serves: 1

**Ingredients:**

- 1 cup unsweetened almond milk or coconut milk
- 1/2 teaspoon ground turmeric
- 1/4 teaspoon ground cinnamon

- 1/4 teaspoon ground ginger
- 1/4 teaspoon honey or maple syrup
- Pinch of black pepper (optional)

**Directions:**

1. In a small saucepan, heat the almond milk or coconut milk over medium heat until hot but not boiling.
2. Add the ground turmeric, ground cinnamon, ground ginger, honey or maple syrup, and black pepper (if using).
3. Whisk the mixture until well combined and heated through.
4. Remove from heat and pour the golden milk into a mug.
5. Allow it to cool slightly before enjoying the warm and comforting anti-inflammatory golden milk.

**Nutritional Value per Serving:**

Calories: 80

Protein: 1g

Fat: 5g

Carbohydrates: 8g

Fiber: 1g

**Recipe 3: Herbal Tea Infusions**

Prep Time: 5 minutes

Steep Time: Varies

Serves: 1

**Ingredients:**

- 1 herbal tea bag (options: chamomile, peppermint, hibiscus, lavender, etc.)
- 1 cup boiling water
- Optional: honey or lemon to taste

**Directions:**

1. Place the herbal tea bag in a cup or mug.
2. Pour boiling water over the tea bag.
3. Let the tea steep for the recommended time on the package instructions (varies depending on the type of herbal tea).

4. Once steeped, remove the tea bag and discard.
5. If desired, sweeten the tea with honey or add a squeeze of lemon for extra flavor.
6. Enjoy the soothing and aromatic herbal tea infusion as a calming and relaxing beverage.

**Nutritional Value per Serving:**

Calories: 0

Protein: 0g

Fat: 0g

Carbohydrates: 0g

Fiber: 0g

## Recipe 4: Ginger Lemonade

Prep Time: 10 minutes

Chill Time: 1 hour

Serves: 4

**Ingredients:**

- 4 cups water
- 1/4 cup freshly squeezed lemon juice
- 2 tablespoons grated ginger
- 2 tablespoons honey or maple syrup
- Optional: lemon slices and mint leaves for garnish

**Directions:**

1. In a saucepan, bring the water to a boil.
2. Add the grated ginger and simmer for 5 minutes.
3. Remove from heat and let it cool slightly.
4. Strain the ginger-infused water into a pitcher.
5. Add the freshly squeezed lemon juice and honey or maple syrup to the pitcher.
6. Stir well to combine.
7. Cover and refrigerate for at least 1 hour to chill and allow the flavors to meld.
8. Serve the ginger lemonade over ice, garnished with lemon slices and mint leaves if desired.
9. Enjoy this refreshing and tangy ginger lemonade as a hydrating and revitalizing drink.

**Nutritional Value per Serving:**

Calories: 35

Protein: 0g

Fat: 0g

Carbohydrates: 9g

Fiber: 0g

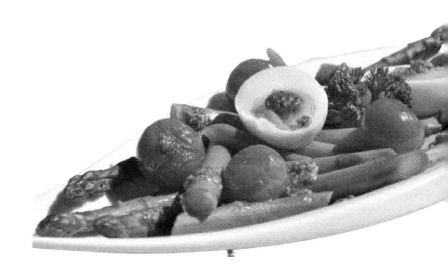

GREEN ASPARAGUS

# CHAPTER 3

## 7-Day Meal Plan for Autoimmune Hepatitis Diet Recipes

### Day 1:

Breakfast:

- Quinoa Breakfast Bowl: Cooked quinoa topped with fresh berries, sliced almonds, and a drizzle of honey.
- Herbal Tea: Enjoy a cup of herbal tea, such as chamomile or ginger, for added antioxidants.

Lunch:

- Grilled Chicken Salad: Grilled chicken breast on a bed of mixed greens, cherry tomatoes, cucumber slices, and a light vinaigrette dressing.
- Steamed Broccoli: Served as a side dish to add extra fiber and nutrients.

Snack:

- Carrot Sticks with Hummus: Enjoy raw carrot sticks with a side of homemade hummus for a healthy and satisfying snack.Dinner:

- Baked Salmon: Oven-baked salmon fillet seasoned with herbs and lemon juice.
- Roasted Sweet Potatoes: Roasted sweet potato wedges seasoned with olive oil, garlic, and paprika.
- Sautéed Spinach: Fresh spinach sautéed with garlic and olive oil.

Day 2:

Breakfast:

- Oatmeal with Berries: Cooked oats topped with mixed berries, chopped walnuts, and a sprinkle of cinnamon.
- Green Tea: Sip on a cup of green tea for added antioxidants.

Lunch:

- Turkey Lettuce Wraps: Lean ground turkey cooked with onions, garlic, and spices, served in lettuce cups with shredded carrots and cucumber.
- Cabbage Slaw: Freshly shredded cabbage mixed with grated carrots, dressed with a light vinaigrette.

Snack:

- Apple Slices with Almond Butter: Enjoy crisp apple slices with a dollop of almond butter for a satisfying snack.

Dinner:

- Grilled Chicken Breast: Grilled chicken breast seasoned with herbs and served with a side of steamed asparagus.
- Quinoa Pilaf: Quinoa cooked with sautéed onions, bell peppers, and diced tomatoes.

Day 3:

Breakfast:

- Veggie Omelette: A fluffy omelette made with egg whites, filled with sautéed spinach, mushrooms, and diced tomatoes.
- Herbal Tea: Enjoy a cup of herbal tea, such as peppermint or lemon verbena, for a refreshing start to the day.

Lunch:

- Lentil Soup: Hearty lentil soup made with vegetables, herbs, and spices.
- Mixed Green Salad: A side salad with mixed greens, cherry tomatoes, cucumber slices, and a light dressing.

Snack:

- Greek Yogurt with Berries: Creamy Greek yogurt topped with fresh berries and a sprinkle of granola.

Dinner:

- Baked Cod: Oven-baked cod fillet seasoned with lemon juice, herbs, and a drizzle of olive oil.
- Steamed Green Beans: Fresh green beans steamed until tender and lightly seasoned with salt and pepper.
- Brown Rice: Nutritious brown rice served as a side dish.

**Day 4:**

Breakfast:

- Smoothie Bowl: A refreshing smoothie made with frozen berries, almond milk, spinach, and topped with sliced banana and chia seeds.
- Green Tea: Sip on a cup of green tea for added antioxidants.

Lunch:

- Quinoa Salad: Cooked quinoa mixed with diced cucumbers, cherry tomatoes, diced bell peppers, fresh herbs, and a lemon vinaigrette.
- Roasted Brussels Sprouts: Brussels sprouts roasted with olive oil, garlic, and a sprinkle of sea salt.

Snack:

- Celery Sticks with Almond Butter: Enjoy crunchy celery sticks with a spread of almond butter for a satisfying snack.

Dinner:

- Grilled Shrimp Skewers: Skewered shrimp marinated in a garlic and lemon marinade, grilled to perfection.

- Cauliflower Rice: Grated cauliflower sautéed with onions, garlic, and herbs as a low-carb rice alternative.

- Steamed Asparagus: Tender asparagus spears lightly steamed and seasoned with lemon juice.

## Day 5:

Breakfast:

- Chia Seed Pudding: Chia seeds soaked in almond milk overnight, topped with sliced bananas, chopped nuts, and a drizzle of honey.

- Herbal Tea: Enjoy a cup of herbal tea, such as hibiscus or lavender, for a calming effect.

Lunch:

- Spinach Salad with Grilled Chicken: Fresh spinach leaves topped with grilled chicken, cherry tomatoes, sliced almonds, and a light vinaigrette dressing.

- Roasted Beets: Beets roasted until tender and served as a side dish.

Snack:

- Rice Cakes with Avocado: Crispy rice cakes topped with mashed avocado and a sprinkle of sea salt.

Dinner:

- Baked Turkey Meatballs: Lean ground turkey meatballs baked in a tomato sauce.
- Zucchini Noodles: Spiralized zucchini cooked in a garlic and olive oil sauce.
- Steamed Broccoli: Served as a side dish to add extra fiber and nutrients.

Day 6:
Breakfast:

- Greek Yogurt Parfait: Layered Greek yogurt, granola, and mixed berries for a delicious and protein-packed breakfast.
- Green Tea: Sip on a cup of green tea for added antioxidants.

Lunch:

- Quinoa Stuffed Bell Peppers: Bell peppers stuffed with a mixture of cooked quinoa, sautéed vegetables, and lean ground turkey.
- Mixed Green Salad: A side salad with mixed greens, cherry tomatoes, cucumber slices, and a light dressing.

Snack:

- Sliced Oranges: Enjoy juicy slices of oranges for a refreshing snack.

Dinner:

- Baked Chicken Breast: Oven-baked chicken breast seasoned with herbs and lemon juice.
- Mashed Cauliflower: Steamed cauliflower mashed with garlic, olive oil, and a sprinkle of herbs.
- Steamed Green Beans: Fresh green beans steamed until tender and lightly seasoned with salt and pepper.

**Day 7:**

Breakfast:

- Vegetable Frittata: A flavorful frittata made with egg whites, loaded with sautéed vegetables like bell peppers, onions, and mushrooms.

- Herbal Tea: Enjoy a cup of herbal tea, such as ginger or turmeric, for added antioxidants.

Lunch:

- Tuna Salad Lettuce Wraps: Canned tuna mixed with diced celery, onions, and a light vinaigrette, served in lettuce wraps.

- Cucumber Salad: Sliced cucumbers dressed with lemon juice, olive oil, and a sprinkle of fresh dill.

Snack:

- Trail Mix: A homemade mix of unsalted nuts, seeds, and dried fruits for a nutritious and energizing snack.

Dinner:

- Baked Salmon: Oven-baked salmon fillet seasoned with herbs and a squeeze of fresh lemon juice.

- Roasted Root Vegetables: A medley of roasted root vegetables like carrots, parsnips, and sweet potatoes.
- Sautéed Kale: Fresh kale leaves sautéed with garlic and olive oil.

Remember to adjust portion sizes according to your dietary needs and consult with a healthcare professional or registered dietitian for personalized advice and any specific dietary restrictions. Enjoy these delicious and nutritious meals as part of your autoimmune hepatitis diet.

# CHAPTER 4

## Conclusion

### A. Recap of the Importance of Diet in Autoimmune Hepatitis

Throughout this cookbook, we have emphasized the crucial role that diet plays in managing autoimmune hepatitis. The foods we consume have the power to impact our overall health, and for individuals with autoimmune hepatitis, making mindful dietary choices can significantly contribute to symptom management and liver health.

By focusing on nutrient-dense foods, incorporating anti-inflammatory ingredients, and following the general dietary guidelines provided, you can support your body's immune system, reduce inflammation, and promote liver function. Remember to prioritize whole foods, lean proteins, healthy fats, and a variety of fruits and vegetables in your meals. Additionally, it is vital to limit processed foods, refined sugars, and excessive salt intake, as they can exacerbate inflammation and strain the liver.

B. Encouragement for Exploring and Enjoying Nutritious Recipes

We hope that the recipes in this cookbook have inspired you to embark on a culinary journey filled with delicious and nutritious meals. Eating well does not have to be boring or restrictive. Instead, it can be an opportunity for exploration, creativity, and enjoyment. We encourage you to experiment with the recipes provided, adapting them to your personal taste preferences and dietary needs.

Remember to approach your meals with gratitude and mindfulness. Engage your senses as you savor the flavors, textures, and aromas of each dish. Eating mindfully allows you to fully appreciate the nourishment you are providing to your body and can enhance your overall dining experience.

C. Final Thoughts and Resources for Further Information

As you continue your journey towards managing autoimmune hepatitis through diet, it is essential to seek ongoing support and guidance from healthcare professionals. Consulting with a registered dietitian or nutritionist who specializes in autoimmune conditions can provide personalized recommendations and ensure that your dietary choices align with your specific needs.

Additionally, there are numerous resources available that can further deepen your understanding of autoimmune hepatitis and its connection to diet. Books, websites, and support groups dedicated to liver health and autoimmune conditions can provide valuable information and a sense of community.

Remember, you are not alone in this journey. Reach out to your healthcare team, connect with others who share similar experiences, and continue to educate yourself about the latest research and developments in autoimmune hepatitis.

In conclusion, the Autoimmune Hepatitis Diet Cookbook aims to empower you to take control of your health and well-being through the foods you choose to nourish your body. By embracing a balanced and nutritious diet, you can support your liver, reduce inflammation, and optimize your overall health.

May these recipes bring you joy, satisfaction, and a renewed sense of vitality. Remember, each meal is an opportunity to nourish your body and embrace a lifestyle that supports your well-being. Here's to your health and happiness!

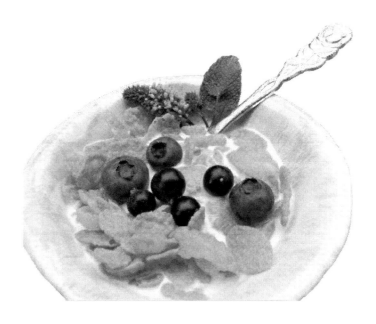

CORN-FLAKES, MILK & BERRY

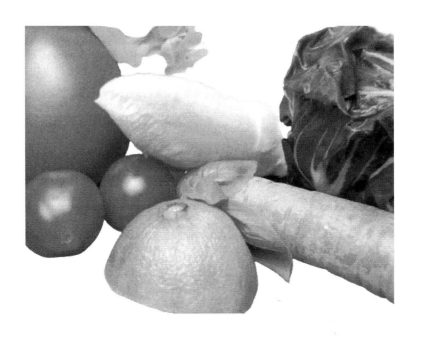

VEGETABLES AND LEMON